FRAN LAKEMAN

EXPECTING BETTER

**The Complete Guide to Pregnancy Philosophy,
Learn All About The Important Facts Surrounding
Pregnancy That You Should Know**

Descrierea CIP a Bibliotecii Naționale a României
FRAN LAKEMAN
    EXPECTING BETTER. The Essential Guide to Mastering Body Language, Learn How to Read and Make Body Movements That Could Pave Your Way to Succes / Fran Lakeman – Bucharest: Editura My Ebook, 2021
    ISBN

FRAN LAKEMAN

EXPECTING BETTER

**The Complete Guide to Pregnancy Philosophy,
Learn All About The Important Facts Surrounding
Pregnancy That You Should Know**

My Ebook Publishing House
Bucharest, 2021

TABLE OF CONTENT

INTRODUCTORY

The first step of your pregnancy, after seeing the little positive stickshould to have it confirmed.

Call immediately to have a pregnancy test done with your local doctor, you may be in luck and get in that same day or have to wait about a week or two. Patience will become your best friend during this time or your worst enemy, waiting can become a very hard thing when you want to know for sure whether you are or aren't pregnant. More than likely you'll get a phonecall a few days later to confirm it.

Set up an appointment to see your OB/GYN or midwife as soon as possible, chances are you'll be meeting his/her staff before you ever meet them. This is the first appointment where your doctor/midwife will want to know all yourmedical history.

If you've been pregnant, what types of sicknesses run in your family, etc. If you can, try making sure you know all of this ahead of time, maybe even have it all down on paper so when he/she asks you are prepared. During the days or weeks leading up to this meeting you may have concerns, write them down and ask them. Believe it or not doctors are there to help you, and they've been asked every question you can possibly think of. Before leaving your doctor may even give you a bag full of goodies all about being pregnant.

Read these, they may prove beneficial and not to mention they've got coupons. Your doctor will either give you another appointment or have you set one up before leaving. There are some great books out there if you are really worried about what will happen next or how birth is going to be, check them out at your local library.

Make sure that you get your prenatal vitamins, they are very important during pregnancy. If for some reason you can't take them, talk with your doctor he/she may be able to prescribe a lower dosage or something else. You'll get your first ultrasound, also known as US around week 20, this is normally when you find out what sex the baby is. However, some doctors like to call it safe and give you an ultrasound around 10-12 weeks just to make sure the baby is in the proper location and all is going well. You will also be asked to take an orange drink that you must drink in five minutes. You'll wait around for an hour to three hours, at which point your blood getsdrawn and you can go home. The test determines if you have or have a chance of getting gestational diabetes.

At first your appointments will be about 4 weeks apart until you hit the 36 weeks and at that point it'll be two weeks later and a week later after that until the baby is born. By now you should be preparing to have the baby. Yes, I'm sure you'll have some anxiety towards the end of your pregnancy. You've went this far, it's time you see your reward.

CHAPTER 1

EXERCISE AND PREGNANCY

Prescribing a medication for pregnant women is a complex process.

Before obstetricians and gynecologists decide which dose of which drug can best treat a condition without putting any harmful side effects on the mother and the baby, they consider the patient's age, general health, the number of months before delivery, tolerance for medications, and any other drugs the pregnant patient may be taking.

Prescribing exercise on pregnant women has to be just as scientific and precise. The type, intensity, frequency, and duration of a "dose" of exercise are all critical. One person's healthy, vigorous workout could be hazardous to another. These dangers may be greater in pregnant women because they are more likely to have strains and other serious side effects for the would be mother.

However, if exercise will be implemented and carried out in a normal, average range, exercise will not have an effect on the overall condition ofthe pregnancy and especially on labor or delivery. Pregnancy

Quality prenatal care should be given to a mother during her pregnancy. Sheshould be prepared for the normal delivery of a healthy baby. Complications should be prevented at all costs.

All of these things are boiled down to the fact that a pregnant woman shouldbe cared in such a way that she will not be compelled to do vigorous work but should not also stay in bed and be inactive until she gives birth to her baby.

Consequently, a pregnant woman's condition varies in relation to the growth and development of the baby inside her womb. Therefore, it is necessary that proper health guidance be provided by her physician during her visit.

Moreover, it is important to keep the pregnant woman's life active in orderto promote good health, not only for her but also for the baby most importantly.

Physical conditions like blood pressure, weight and health status is usually monitored during the pregnant woman's visit to her doctor. For this reason,it is significant to note that exercise can be the number one factor in order to keep these aspects in good condition.

As the health experts contend, adequate physical and emotional informationis needed by a pregnant woman to prepare herself for delivery. She needs practical health messages in keeping herself and the baby healthy.

Hence, for mothers or would-be mothers who are not yet aware why they should exert some effort in engaging into moderate, normal exercise, here isa list of some of its benefits so that you will be able to understand the reason why pregnant women have to exercise regularly:

1. Defiance against fatigue

As muscle becomes fatigued, it produces less force. To accomplish a task like climbing the stairs, for example, or shoveling snow, more units of muscle must be called into play to back up the wearied muscles.

The tired muscles are both less efficient and less effective. Hence, this will just put more strain on the pregnant woman because of the weight that iscontinuously adding up each day. That is why tired muscles will usually result to leg cramps or sore muscles.

What every pregnant woman must know is that exercise improves the condition of the muscles and their ability to work longer without fatigue.

2. Reduce backaches

Even when you sit or stand, some muscles are working, and such relatively easy postures can tax some muscles and cause fatigue. The muscles of the lower back, for example, can be exhausted and worn out by the effort of keeping erect when a pregnant woman stand still for several hours.

With exercise, a pregnant woman can correct this error by developing herposture.

3. Increase the amount of oxygen

Work and exercise rely on glycogen, a substance produced by the body fromcomplex carbohydrates and stored muscles and liver. The supply of glycogen in the muscles determines and limits the duration of activity. Exercise depletes the glycogen in the muscles and leads to tiredness.

However, when glycogen is depleted by strenuous activity, it is replaced in quantities greater than before, as if the body recognized the need to lay in alarger supply of fuel.

Hence, oxidation is essential for converting glycogen to the energy that pregnant women need to wiggle a finger, flex a muscle, or practice the lungs and heart for some blowing action during normal delivery.

These are just some of the many benefits exercise can bring to pregnant women. Besides, nothing is completely wrong for a pregnant woman doing some moderate exercises. The only important thing to remember is that before starting an exercise program, whether pregnant or not, it is best to consult your doctor. As they say, doctors know best!

CHAPTER 2

FOOD CRAVINGS DURINGPREGNANCY

Do pickles and ice cream sound good to you? How about redpeppers and peanut butter?

If these do, you are probably a pregnant woman who has just gone looking for that ice cream carton you know you have buried in your freezer. More than three quarters of all pregnant women experience cravings at some point.

The most common cravings are for sweets, dairy products and salty foods although there are some weird cravings out there. Some women have been known to put black olives on cheesecake, while others have been known to dip fruit in salsa. As bizarre as some cravings can be, they are mainly perfectly safe.

There are old wife's tales that believe what you crave could be a good indication of the sex of your baby. If you are craving sweets you are having a girl. If you crave meats or cheeses, it is believed you are having a boy.

Cravings are something that most women love most about pregnancy. It is when a woman is craving dirt or clay that an alarm should go off.

If you should find yourself craving dirt, soil, or chalk call your doctor right away. Not only could these be harmful if you do eat them, but chances are they are a sign of iron-deficiency anemia.

Most doctors believe that cravings can be nutritionally based. That is to say the cravings are a message from your body on what it needs to eat. If you are craving salts foods it could be because your body needs more sodium as your blood volume increases. If you are craving fruit, your body might need more vitamins C.

The problem is sometimes the message gets lost on the way to our brain. You may find yourself craving something sweet and instead of getting berries or fruit, you find yourself gulping down snicker bars by the cart full. Cravings can be the downfall of your weight gain especially if the message is getting scrambled. There are some ways though you can help curb your cravings.

For starters, eat a good breakfast. Eating a good breakfast can prevent cravings later in the day. You also want to try and make wise choices by looking for healthier alternatives. If you are dying for potato chips try eating some soy crisps. Instead of ice cream, try frozen yogurt. If you feel like candy is calling your name, snack on some frozen grapes. If you want something salty try pretzels, or even rice cakes to satisfy that urge. A good substation for soda would be some fruit juice mixed with sparkling water.

Next, think small. If you are craving chocolate, you do no need to reach for a king size bar. The snack size bar will satisfy your craving just the same. If you want a brownie, have one; just do not eat the whole pan. There is nothing wrong with indulging in a few of your cravings as long as you know not to overdo it.

Giving in to your cravings during pregnancy does not make you a bad person and it is not something you should beat yourself up about and feel guilty about. Cravings are a normal part of pregnancy and denying yourself all the time might make you resent being pregnant. Indulge when you want to, just make sure you make wise choices and do everything in moderation.

CHAPTER 3

UNPLANNED PREGNANCIES

Pregnancy is often a pleasant surprise. Of course, there are timesthat pregnancy can come as a shock.

Although most unplanned pregnancies are still pleasant surprises, it doesn't make the situation much easier. There are steps you can take to make an unplanned pregnancy a pleasant experience.

First, speak with a friend or family member you can trust. You'll need someone who will be supportive and not condescending. It's already an emotional time for you. The last thing you need is the added stress of defending the pregnancy.

Second, once you're past the initial stages of finding out about your pregnancy, prepare yourself for the varying responses of other people. You may get receptions that are congratulatory, and you may get some who are judgmental. Be prepared for both. Also remember that what's done is done. It's not constructive to look back in regret, anger, or despair. It is better to look forward and to make the best of the surprise situation.

Third, don't feel as if you're alone. Unplanned pregnancies happen to many people. There are support groups both online and offline available to help you through this confusing time in your life. Seek their counsel. Don't be afraid to voice your own fears and concerns. You may find the sessions verytherapeutic.

Fourth, prepare to inform the baby's father. Obviously, it won't be easy, andyou'll get a varying range of responses from excitement to denial. Hopefully,the father will be supportive and can help you through the pregnancy.

Fifth, be aware that your body is in a different state. Because you're now pregnant, your body is flooded with hormones and is transforming every day. Take this into account when talking with people and prioritizing yourlife.

Induced Abortion

Induced abortion is the deliberate termination of pregnancy in a manner that ensures that the embryo or fetus will not survive. Attitudes of society toward elective abortion have undergone marked changes in the past few decades.

In some situations, the need for abortion is accepted by most people, but political and medical attitudes regarding induced abortion have continued to lag behind changing philosophies. Some religious concepts remain unchanged, resulting in personal, medical, and political conflicts.

About one-third of the world's population lives in nations with nonrestrictivelaws governing abortion. Another third live in countries with moderately restrictive abortion laws, i.e., where unwanted pregnancies may not be terminated as a matter of right or personal decision but only on broadly interpreted medical, psychologic, and sociologic indications.

The remainder live in countries where abortion is illegal without qualification or is allowed only when the woman's life or health would be severely threatened if the pregnancy were allowed to continue.

An estimated 1 out of every 4 pregnancies in the world is terminated by induced abortion, making it perhaps the most common method of reproduction limitation. In the U.S., estimates of the number of criminal abortions performed prior to legalization of the procedure ranged from 0.25-1.25 million per year.

The number of legal abortions now being performed in this country approximates 1 abortion per 4 live births. In 1997, there were 1.33 million induced abortions compared to 3.88 million live births.

Legal Aspects of Induced Abortion in the United States

The United States Supreme Court ruled in 1973 (1) that the restrictive abortion laws in the U.S. were invalid, largely because these laws invaded the individual's right to privacy, and (2) that an abortion could not be denied to a woman in the first 3 months of pregnancy.

The Court indicated that after 3 months a state may "regulate the abortion procedure in ways that are reasonably related to maternal health" and that after the fetus reaches the stage of viability (about 24 weeks) the states may refuse the right to terminate the pregnancy except when necessary for the preservation of the life or health of the mother.

Still, much opposition is raised by various "right-to-life" groups and religious groups. In spite of this opposition, over 1 million procedures are still performed annually in the United States, with about one-third being performed on teenaged women.

This dramatically emphasizes the inadequacy of sex education and the need for greater availability of adequate contraceptive methods in order to avoid such pregnancy wastage.

Evaluation of Patients Requesting Induced Abortion

Patients give varied reasons for requesting abortion. Since in some cases the request is made at the urging of the woman's parents or in-laws, husband, or peers, every effort should be made to ascertain that the patient herself desires abortion for her own reasons. In addition, one should be certain that she knows she is free to choose among other methods of solving the problem of unplanned pregnancy, e.g., adoption or single-parent rearing.

Although the majority of abortions are performed as elective procedures, i.e., because of social or economic reasons as opposed to medical reasons, some women still request such services for medical or surgical indications.

For example, for women with certain medical conditions, such as

Eisenmenger's complex and cystic fibrosis, continuation of pregnancy may pose a threat to the life of the mother. Other indications are pregnancy resulting from a rape or pregnancy with a fetus affected with a major disorder, e.g., trisomy 13. In any event, the ultimate decision rests with the pregnant woman.

CHAPTER 4

OVULATION

Childbirth is a momentous occasion, whether a first born or theseventh.

The health and upbringing of a newborn is dependent on mother's preparedness on how she handles this delicate issue. We can read or watch videos of childbirth but it is experience that carries weight.

The first step is to understand female anatomy and how it works during different phases of childbirth. Ovulation is one such phase of the menstrual cycle, when an egg or ovum is released from ovaries. If this ovum meets with male sperm in its journey down the fallopian tube conception takes place. It does sound simple, but Ovulation depends on the interplay of glands and hormones.

This may be one reason why some women cannot conceive. The gland that affects Ovulation is the Hypothalamus, using its hormones for communication with the pituitary gland, referred to as the master gland of the endocrine system. In turn, the pituitary gland produces luteinizing hormone (LH) and FSH. High levels of LH cause Ovulation within two days.

The cycle continues with mature follicles releasing ovum into the peritoneal cavity and then into the fallopian tube, and from there to the uterus. If the ovum does not encounter a sperm within 24 hours it dies.

Ovulation occurs two weeks before the onset of the menstrual period once every month till menopause, or break in between for child birth and pregnancy. Certain changes occur in the cervical mucus, which gets slippery and slick, accompanied by general or localized pain. Sometimes there is delay or deviation from 24 to 35 days in the menstrual cycle, or slight fever in women who follow natural family planning methods.

This persuades them to mistake Ovulation for premenstrual symptoms, if accompanied by pain and changes in body. Instead of playing guessing games, Ovulation should be confirmed with kits available in market or through blood tests or pregnancy ultrasound. Once sure, it is advisable to take precautions to avoid miscarriage or bleeding. Motherhood is something nature intended us to enjoy, and we should welcome it in all its cycles.

CHAPTER 5

OVERCOMING THE PAIN
OF AFAILED PREGNANCY

Imagine a newlywed couple eager to have their first baby. After months of anticipation and careful attention to the pregnancy, the unexpected happens --- they suffer a miscarriage.

The trauma of losing an unborn child is a difficult period for any couple, but more so for the would-be first-time mother. After miscarriage and other forms of pregnancy loss, most couples usually have a lot of questions that need to be answered. A lot of people take it upon themselves to answer why the miscarriage happened and exactly how they could have prevented pregnancy.

But usually, miscarriage is rarely anyone's fault, and sometimes pregnancy loss is even a predetermined outcome at the time of conception. There may not be any explanation at hand why miscarriages happen, though, the medical community recognizes a few known miscarriage causes. A number of theories abound regarding the cause of miscarriage.

One-time pregnancy loss, also called sporadic, are usually caused by chromosomal abnormalities while the fetus develops. A lot of times, doctorsassume this as the default explanation for first time miscarriages due to thefact that most couples go on to have a normal pregnancy after one miscarriage.

Chromosomal abnormalities such as extra chromosomes or missing genes may cause the baby to stop developing and eventually to be miscarried.

After the first miscarriage, most medical professionals do not conduct testing for the cause of miscarriage since chromosomal flaws are usually random, one-time events. Miscarriage due to chromosomal flaws may occur to any woman at any age, but those who are 35 years old and above are at highestrisk.

When a miscarriage happens two times in a row, the cause is unlikely to be random chromosomal errors in a row. Usually, doctors will conduct a process of testing for recurrent miscarriage causes after the second pregnancy loss.

In this case, chances are higher that the woman may have a detectableproblem that causes the miscarriage.

About 50% of the cases, doctors find a cause for recurrent miscarriages and then the woman is given treatment in her next pregnancy. However, half of the cases may not reveal a cause. At any rate, a woman may still get pregnant again even with two unexplained miscarriages, and still with greater chances of a normal pregnancy than another miscarriage.

Causes of recurrent miscarriages are usually much more controversialcompared to that of single miscarriages.

The following is a list of some of the most commonly recognizedcauses of recurrent miscarriages:

- Abnormality in the structure of the uterus.
- Blood clotting disorders, such as antiphospholipid syndrome.
- Certain chromosomal conditions, such as balanced translocation.

Doctors believe that low progesterone and other hormonal imbalances may cause recurrent miscarriages. Although treatment with progesterone supplements is fairly common after one or two pregnancy losses, however, not all medical practitioners agree on the practice. Others believe that malfunction in the immune system, such as high levels of natural killer cells,may be the culprit.

Pregnancy losses after the 20th week are called stillbirths. Too-early births, on the other hand, are called preterm labors. Both preterm labors and stillbirths usually have different causes from earlier miscarriages, although chromosomal errors in the baby can also cause stillbirths.

The most common causes of stillbirths and preterm labors are cervical insufficiency, problems in the placenta, and preterm labor due to medicalissues in the mother.

No matter what may be the cause of pregnancy loss, the woman is advised to seek out emotional support from friends and relatives. Counseling helps a lot in dealing with the emotional aftermath of miscarriage.

CHAPTER 6

MAKE YOUR PREGNANCY AHEALTHY ONE

Congratulations! You're pregnant! Now, let's get down to business.

According to the National Women's Health Resource Center (NWHRC), everything you do in the next nine months, from what you eat to what you drink to how physically active you are and what you weigh, has the potential to affect your child's current and future growth.

In fact, a new report by NWHRC explores the growing body of research thatfinds conditions in utero (i.e., while you're pregnant) have the potential to affect your child's health even decades down the road.

For instance, one study found that women who drink during pregnancy could increase their child's risk of alcohol addiction later in life, even with just one drinking binge. Other studies suggest significant correlations between a mother's nutrition during pregnancy and her child's risk for being overweight and developing diabetes and heart disease later in life.

The message? Eat right today and prevent future health problems for yourchild.

There are two components to "eating right" when you're pregnant. One is the type of food you're eating, and the other is how much weight you gain.

For many women, pregnancy is the first time in their lives when gaining weight is a good thing-but don't go overboard. You do not need to consumeany more calories than your normal daily intake during your first trimester. After the first 12 weeks, you may consume up to 300 extra calories per day.

If you are of normal weight when you get pregnant, you should gain between 25 and 35 pounds. Limit weight gain to no more than five to 10 pounds in the first 20 weeks, and about a pound per week for the remainderof your pregnancy.

Doctors strongly suggest, however, that if you are overweight, to try and lose some weight before you get pregnant. Women who are overweight have a higher risk of emergency cesarean, gestational diabetes, high blood pressure and miscarriage. There is also a greater risk of delivery complications.

Your health care professional will help you determine where you fall on theweight scale during your first prenatal visit.

As always, talk to your health care professional about any special dietary concerns (if you're vegetarian or vegan, for example).

CHAPTER 7

LOSING WEIGHT AFTERPREGNANCY

You could be lucky. I was - just once. When my middle daughter was born I actually weighed 10 pounds less than I had when I'd conceived her.

That's not something you can count on, though, and I can tell you that from experience as well. Most women start their lives as a new mom with an extra 8 to 15 pounds that they didn't have pre-baby.

There's a very good reason for that. God designed our bodies with nurture in mind. Part of that weight that you put on during pregnancy was meant to nurture your baby AFTER birth.

While your body requires an extra 300 calories a day to keep up with the nutritional demands of your baby during pregnancy, a breastfeeding mother requires at least 500 extra calories a day to produce enough milk and remain healthy. Your body stores up a little extra nutrition for after the birthjust in case there isn't enough food for its needs when it's time to feed the new little critter.

If you're breastfeeding, that's part of the good news. You'll automatically be burning an extra five hundred calories a day - which will make it considerably easier for you to lose the extra weight. In fact, you may not need to do anything special at all to lose weight.

Just focus on eating a normal, healthy, well-balanced diet. If you're not breastfeeding, you won't find it quite as easy. Your focus should still be onhealthy eating, with moderate exercise to burn extra calories.

Here's more good news for new mothers. Exercising is easier. Actually, that's not quite right. Burning more calories is easier. Walking alone for an hour burns 200 calories. Walking while pushing a stroller ups that figure considerably. Push a stroller uphill, and it's even higher.

You'll get extra duty out of things you never thought of like lifting the strollerand car seat in and out of the car, carrying the baby up and down stairs and just plain carrying the baby.

Still. If you find yourself with stubborn pounds that simply won't come off,exercise and a moderate reduction in calories is the way to go. Just like pregnancy isn't the time for weight loss, just after pregnancy isn't the timeto stress your body further with severe dietary restrictions.

Aim for losing about a pound a week, though chances are you'll find it coming off faster than that. Being a mom is a high-energy proposition!

CHAPTER 8

KNOW THE EARLY SIGNS OFPREGNANCY

I'm pregnant? How can that be? I was not expecting this to happen!

These are some of the common reactions of women who became aware of their pregnancy at the very last moment. Since many women today basically missed the early signs of pregnancy, they only became aware that they are indeed pregnant after they try using a home pregnancy kit or after their gynecologists confirm it.

To avoid the hassle and drama of unwanted pregnancy, it is best for all sexually active women to become responsible enough to engage in safe sexand of course, to become aware of the early signs of pregnancy.

The following are the seven signs of pregnancy:

1. Light to moderate spotting

Moderate spotting generally occurs before a woman's menstrual period begins. Spotting can also be a sign of pregnancy as implantation starts. Since this type of bleeding is brownish and the flow is usually light to moderate just like the pre-menstrual spotting, some women often disregard it as an early sign of pregnancy.

2. Increased body temperature

Just like the spotting, sudden increased in body temperature is also one of the most frequently missed signs of pregnancy among women, for this also normally happens during menstrual period. If a woman's basal body temperature is higher than normal, then it can be a symptom for pregnancy.

3. Nausea

Nausea or morning sickness is one of the most common signs of pregnancy.This basically happens during the first to two weeks of pregnancy. Although the feeling of nausea and vomiting oftentimes occur anytime within the day, these can trigger when one least expects it.

4. Missed period

A missed period is probably the most obvious indication that a woman is pregnant. When this happens, women tend to immediately look for other signs of pregnancy or better yet, confirm their condition by means of reliablepregnancy home kit.

5. Frequent urination

A pregnant woman may not notice her frequent trips to the comfort room, but others can easily notice this, thus, an indication of pregnancy. This symptom happens because the uterus begins to swell and pressure on the bladder eventually occurs.

6. Tender breasts and nipples

Tender and swollen breasts and nipples are signs of menstrual bleeding, but these can also be indications that a woman might be pregnant. A woman may notice such soreness during sleeping, exercising, and even while getting dressed. Apart from soreness and tenderness of the breast as possible signs of pregnancy, a woman may also notice that her nipples darken in color.

7. Exhaustion or fatigue

A sudden feeling of fatigue or exhaustion is also one of the early signs of pregnancy. A woman can tell if she's pregnant when she easily becomes exhausted and tired even after doing little or no activity at all.

These are just seven of the many early signs of pregnancy. Since the symptoms explained above are perhaps the most obvious indications that a woman is pregnant, one should confirm pregnancy by immediately consulting a gynecologist. Keep in mind that not all signs of pregnancy apply to every woman, hence, a trip to the gynae can definitely save one from theparanoia of possible pregnancy.

Printed by Libri Plureos GmbH in Hamburg,
Germany